Anxiety

Keys to leaving anxiety behind

Peter Michell

Introduction

Anxiety can vary from relatively mild to totally devastating. At one level the adrenalin it produces has an important part to play in keeping us safe from danger – at another level it can ruin people's lives, cause extreme physical pain sometimes leading to self-harm and suicidal thoughts, and worse, even suicide.

In this booklet we will learn about how it works and develops and how to overcome it. The study will cover the 'natural' causes and effects and will bring in the biblical aspect.

The study comes from experience and gifting – it is my hope that it will be a great help bringing release to those affected.

Christians are to know – if they suffer anxiety, they have *not* failed the Lord God or themselves – rather they are under attack, possibly severe attack. This study, I hope, will help overcome the attack.

All references are from the New King James Bible

Contents

Chapter 1
Tigers

She looked behind her, there was a tiger. Her body responded. Adrenalin flowed, blood oxygen increased. Her body was fully alerted and ready to fight or to flee. She fled – full speed away from the danger.
After about 50 yards she stopped. Where was the tiger? She had expected to be overrun by now. She looked back. It was still in exactly the same position and very still. She watched for a couple of minutes before creeping back towards it. Still no movement at all. She got closer and closer - it still looked ferocious but something was wrong. As she came up to it she saw it was a very lifelike, full size, cardboard cut out tiger. It was just a paper tiger!

Thanks to a local GP for the concept of paper tigers – that came from his extensive experience of dealing with patients suffering from anxiety. (Sometimes known as 'generalised anxiety') Anxiety, he tells us, is full of paper tigers - that is worries and fears with no substance in fact. They appear very realistic and frightening but actually amount to nothing.

The Oxford English dictionary defines anxiety as, 'a nervous disorder marked by excessive uneasiness.'

The Holy Bible says, *'Be anxious for nothing, but in everything by prayer and supplication, with thanksgiving, let your requests be known to God,'* (Philippians 4:6)

As Paul wouldn't be advising the Philippian church to do the impossible. (chapter 4, verse 6) we can conclude – there is a pathway away from excessive uneasiness to becoming anxious for nothing. That would be the fulfilment of Jesus statement that He leaves His peace for us to enjoy. (John 14:27)

Chapter 1 - Notes

Important points:

Most anxiety is caused by 'paper tigers' That is things, fears, which are not true.

Your own notes -

Chapter 2
What causes anxiety

The dictionary definition has already given us a valuable tool -it described anxiety as excessive uneasiness.

In 2020 and 2021 the covid pandemic swept through the world making many very uneasy. Would they succumb to it? How bad would it be? Pictures of hospitals in Italy in particular, overrun by the number of sufferers, filled the television screens.

The UK government (and probably others) panicked and started a campaign of fear by constant pronouncements, lockdowns, restrictions and very unsettling images in the media. Supposed experts made claims wildly exaggerating the likely number of deaths. The government's panic was fuelled by this supposedly expert advice.

As a result the number of people suffering from excessive uneasiness, anxiety, increased hugely.

Anxiety is caused by excessive uneasiness. It doesn't need a pandemic in order to affect many people. The uneasiness can have many sources. Worry about health, about money, about jobs, about relationships and many other matters and even nothing specific can lead to anxiety. These thoughts do not automatically lead to one suffering from anxiety – it will depend on the degree of 'house room' given to them.

The Lord God could, of course, remove anxiety at a stroke – but that would interfere with our freewill as we will see as we progress.

What causes anxiety?

Frequently those who suffer from anxiety jump to the conclusion that there is a medical cause – maybe unbalanced chemical make up in the body or some such thing. And so to the doctor in the hope of medication that will correct the situation.

When one speaks with medical professionals they freely confess that in the vast majority of cases there is no medical cure. They prescribe drugs to soften the effects and that can be helpful but cannot cure the problem. Over time dosages have to increase as the body becomes accustomed to the drugs.

Back to the GP for the concept of paper tigers.

Tigers are dangerous

In our opening story we saw how the girl responded. She perceived danger, meaning something bad was going to happen and she would not be able to cope.

Adrenalin

Then we saw how the body responds to a threat. The tiger was seen and registered as a threat. The body responded by producing adrenalin – the body is designed to do exactly that in order to keep us safe. This is the good effect of adrenalin – it is known to empower us to either fight or flee. (Or sometime faint) Adrenalin has a good part to play. However it can also cause pain and difficulty when produced unnecessarily.

We will see that our thinking plays a very important part – indeed the crucial role

'Danger' perceived in the mind.

Anxiety is described as a mental illness, meaning it is located in one's thinking. The girl thought the tiger she saw was a danger to her and responded accordingly. However, it turned out to be just a realistic looking cut out.

This is the problem. To one who has become sensitive to anxiety, the mind can perceive paper tigers, looking very realistic and causing the body's adrenalin reaction - where actually there is no threat at all.

These 'paper tigers' very realistically look like danger, leading to the thought 'something bad is going to happen' and to 'I won't be able to cope.' These cause the body to feel threatened, to perceive danger and to respond with adrenalin to equip for 'fight or flee.' These worries appear to be very very real to the sufferer but actually amount to nothing.

It is helpful to recognise the reality - these anxious thoughts are 99.9% of the time 'paper tigers.' It's similar to the man in the desert suffering from extreme thirst – he sees an oasis in the distance and with great effort makes his way in that direction only to discover it was a mirage, no water. So it is with 'paper tigers' – no actual danger at all.

Another important area is what we think of ourselves. Here the enemy plants many lies - such as;

I feel guilty, I feel like a failure, I feel inadequate, I feel nobody likes me, I feel I am being punished and any similar self-deprecating thoughts. Our view of our own value is diminished – the body senses danger!

As these are seen by our being as danger adrenalin will be produced and anxiety created or increased. They are certainly lies. Like many lies there be just a grain of truth. Yes we might fail at something, however that does not make us a failure. It just means we are human. Each human is made in the image of God and thus has the potential to become a fruitful member of society

The bible tells us that *as a man thinks, so he is.* So the bible confirms that with anxiety, it is the mind that plays **the** vital role, except in the very rare cases of some other cause. An imbalance in the thyroid gland can be a cause - a blood test will show whether this is relevant or not.

Back to the local GP - in cases of anxiety he won't do blood tests, unless very strongly pushed to do so, as in his experience the need is so very rare.

For the majority of cases it is what we allow our minds to focus on that is the problem. Frequently these things are 'automatic' thoughts. That is our mind responds automatically to a situation.

The KEY realisation ia to acknowledge and understand that the anxious thoughts have no basis in truth - they are not rational.

So we need to learn how to deal with these things.

Looking for alternative causes or roots.

It is often difficult to accept that the negative thoughts and feelings that assail our minds and dwell there, if we let them, are the cause - surly there must be some other cause or root to this problem!
Then there is the temptation to go rooting about trying to find 'the cause or root.' This is very unhelpful and poor counselling can lead us astray.

Simply ask the Holy Spirit to reveal if there is another cause or root or even a spiritual root. Wait for His answer – no answer = no other cause or root. The Holy Spirit is the very best counsellor.

The danger with rooting about in one's past lies in latching on to, or even imagining, all sorts of possibilities. One even hears of people being told the cause or root is things that happened even before birth!

Unless the Holy Spirit has clearly revealed something to you (not others) when you pray, resist rooting about and settle it in your mind - yes, negative thoughts and feelings even thoughts **alone** can be a common cause of anxiety.

(If something is revealed to you by the Holy Spirit you can deal with it in prayer as He leads you.)

Chapter 2 – Notes

Important points

Wrong thinking creates anxiety which causes the body to react producing adrenalin. Beware irrational thoughts.

Your own notes -

Chapter 3
How to deal with its effects.

Anxiety feeds on the perception of danger which is fed by our thinking. At first this may seem unlikely – but there is now a growing awareness that this is indeed the case. Cognitive Behaviour Therapy (CBT) is now a well-established and successful method of treatment.

When one becomes anxious there are practical things which will help.
The first is to control one's breathing. Breathe in to the count of 4, hold it for 2, breathe out to 3 or 4, wait for 2, then breathe in again continuing this process for a few minutes. The anxiety will reduce to some extent.
More severe, very anxious – go for a walk or take other physical exercise. How does this help? It burns off excess blood oxygen produced as a result of the adrenalin response.

Distraction can also help. Though you may not feel like it choose to do something positive, or study or listen to music

Having someone close to help, maybe to count the seconds for breathing, or to accompany on a walk, will definitely assist the sufferer.

These three physical things will help. But much more important is to address one's thinking. All the time negative and threatening things are being turned over in the mind fuel is being pumped into the anxiety, creating more adrenalin - making it worse and worse.

The concept of 'red' and green' thoughts can be helpful. Red stands for danger – don't go there! 'Red' thoughts would be negative, or self-deprecating or assuming the worst or something bad. 'Red' thoughts appear to be dangerous to the soul, increasing uneasiness and anxiety - thereby increasing the flow of adrenalin and as a result increasing 'emotional' pain and discomfort.

A lot of 'red' thoughts start with 'what if' followed by imagining something bad or unhelpful. These are future things which in reality are very unlikely to happen, but cause pain now for no reason. A very helpful thing to do is to 'live in the present,' and not in an imaginary future!

In Chapter 5 is a quotation from the bible which describes what I am calling 'Green' thoughts. These are safe and good

Suffering from anxiety, one can become much more sensitive than usual to any form of negative thinking. So recognising things which act as triggers will help.

Chapter 3 – Notes

Important points

Start to recognise 'red' and 'green' thinking and cut out the 'red' thoughts.

Your own notes -

Chapter 4
Recognising triggers

Let's recognise that for many sufferers the anxiety they experience can or will seem to be totally irrational – there being no obvious reason for it, nothing to worry about. Hence the thinking it must be chemical or medical. But the working of the mind has been overlooked and when suffering anxiety even very small things in the mind can trigger the adrenalin response. Hence anxiety appears irrational.

For instance – ahead is a difficult situation. Maybe a meeting, maybe work related, maybe the result of some unwise action, or whatever. The thought persists – this is going to be difficult, maybe very difficult, probably I won't cope. The thought is not fact - it is speculating what might happen and it can build up into a significant 'paper tiger' very easily.
Being in a sensitised state the one suffering from anxiety is easily upset. Even the simplest thing – like meeting a friend for coffee can be a trigger leading to a manifestation of acute anxiety.

One of the effects sufferers of anxiety experience is 'good days' and 'bad days.' The minor irritations of life are easily brushed off on a good day. On a bad day the same minor incident can set off a serious anxiety attack.

It is like a gun or rifle which are designed to shoot - some have a trigger which requires a firm squeeze to fire the gun, others have what we call a 'hair trigger' - the slightest touch sets of the gun.

Those suffering anxiety are more sensitive – on a 'hair trigger' which even little wrong thoughts can set off. Anxiety seems very irrational and it is.

For those alongside - be aware that over empathising with others, including family members, could cause or increase your own anxiety and is not appropriate. Much better to pray for them – casting all your cares on the Lord Jesus Christ, who is able to actually help them, as we are invited to do.

Anxiety is most frequently worry about what might happen at some future time. The basis is speculation that things will be bad. It could be looked on as living in the future rather than the immediate present. No one knows the future so such negative speculation is totally unhelpful.
Jesus understood – *'Therefore do not worry about tomorrow, for tomorrow will worry about its own things. Sufficient for the day is its own trouble.'* Live for now!   Matthew 6:34

Chapter 4 - Notes

Important points

Recognise the sufferer from anxiety has a heightened
level of sensitivity.

Your own notes -

Chapter 5
The role of the mind in achieving freedom

Consider this analogy – if we compare our minds to a car. The car will run well on good fuel – but put petrol in a diesel engine or diesel in a petrol engine or use contaminated fuel and the car will not run well or even not at all.

My mind and your mind can be said to run on fuel. For the mind, fuel is our thoughts. The wisdom of scripture, whilst telling us to be anxious for nothing, has this advice regarding our thinking in the letter to the Philippians, chapter 4 verse 8: *'Whatever things are true, whatever things are noble, whatever things are just, whatever things are pure, whatever things are lovely, whatever things are of good report, if there is any virtue and if there is anything praiseworthy – meditate on these things.'* This is a definition of 'good fuel!' ('Green' thoughts, from Chapter 3)

On the other hand the common experience with anxiety is to think on worthless things, to think and assume there will be bad things coming our way, and to put ourselves down as inadequate or useless or whatever negative thought comes our way. Often these negative thoughts seem to come automatically. Negative ('red') thoughts are likened to 'bad or contaminated fuel!'

It is helpful to be aware and to change one's thinking at the earliest possible moment – to stop the flow of bad fuel producing more and more adrenalin.

We have already seen that the vast majority of 'bad' thoughts are paper tigers - that is one way of saying they are lies, they are not the truth. They appear very real to the sufferer – the road to freedom starts with the understanding 'these things are lies' and I don't have to think them, they are just paper tigers!

The antidote to lies is the truth.
It is here that the bible believer has a great advantage – God has laid out _the truth_ for us in the scripture.
However, to enjoy this advantage means getting a very sound understanding of the truth. Study and seeking the Holy Spirit to lead us into all truth as we study is very helpful in building us up in the truth.

Rather than just accepting our thoughts and feelings we can apply some rational analysis weakening the lie. Say we are going to undertake a job or activity of some sort. Our thoughts and feelings warn the anxious that it won't work out well or we won't be able to cope. But look rationally, we have done this or similar things before, maybe a lot of times, and it has always worked out well. The thoughts and feelings were just paper tigers – lies.

To the bible believer this can be understood. The scripture tells us there are evil forces at work robbing, killing and destroying. One look at the world demonstrates this is abundantly true. Jesus warned that our enemy, the prince, ruler, of this world was and is a liar from the beginning. Do not be surprised therefore that we suffer from an abundance of lies in this world.

Truth is the antidote to lies.

For sufferers from anxiety a little negative thinking, a little acceptance of the lies, provides fuel and then with danger perceived (even though not real) the body pumps adrenalin.
We need to get over the fact that it doesn't seem rational. When suffering with anxiety it is not rational. In normal health anxiety can be easily dealt with. For one suffering from anxiety it easily escalates becoming emotionally painful – sometimes leading to self -harm, suicidal thoughts and worse.

The recognition that anxiety is, in the vast majority of cases, an issue in the mind and not due to some sort of undiagnosed chemical imbalance, will open the doorway to control thereof and even freedom. That is not to say the pathway is easy – rather it will need to be worked at – but the way through to relief becomes available and in the hands of the sufferer.

There are many 'helps' available on the internet and in books. Here are a few.

NHS Cumbria, Northumberland, Tyne and Wear produce a self-help guide to anxiety (and other things) which can be freely downloaded at www.cntw.nhs.uk/selfhelp

'The feeling good handbook' by David D Burns is excellent. (Available on Amazon.) Number 1 choice!

An introductory self-help course in Cognitive Behaviour Therapy. www.getselfhelp.co.uk

The importance of hope

Believers will know that the bible speaks of hope as very important. One of the effects of anxiety is to reduce, or remove, hope. 'Will I ever recover?' 'How do I get out of this?' and similar thoughts.

The answer is that full recovery back to 'normal' life is entirely possible. Biblically hope has both an eternal and a temporal aspect. Our eternal hope – that of eternity in glory is totally guaranteed. Temporal hope - that is hope in this life, is subject to the statement that we *'work out our own salvation (deliverance from danger) with fear and trembling.* (Philippians 2:12)

Certainly anxiety can be left behinds us as we use the keys outlined herein. It does need to be worked at – it is a process of learning, accepting and applying. There will be 'ups' and 'downs.' For the believer the Lord God will help.

As the scripture puts it, *'Do not cast away your confidence (or hope), which has great reward,'* Hebrews 10:35

Hope helps us win through! When suffering anxiety even fixing hope on some small thing will be helpful – no hope at all is very weakening. A little hope goes a long way! At times of severe stress even reminding oneself that it is not always this bad – it has been better, so it can be better again. And today may have been bad but that does not mean tomorrow will be bad.

Chapter 5 – Notes

Important points-

Recognise lies and distortions are fuel for anxiety

Your own notes -

Chapter 6
The role of prayer

For the believer – we are invited in the scripture to seek the Lord at the throne of grace to find grace and mercy to help in times of need. (Hebrews 4:16) Prayer – that is speaking out one's need to the Lord, is simple. However there may be somethings to overcome.
It is easy to get into the wrong mind set, even for believers – thinking such as:
I am not worthy to pray
God won't answer me
It is hopeless
… and so on.

These are, of course, each and every one, lies.
Every believer has been given the free gift of righteousness (Romans 5:17) - that is 'right standing' with God. You have been made worthy in Christ.
The Lord invites us to pray and express our needs to Him (Hebrews 4:16), so of course He will answer.
The scripture tell us that the thoughts of God, towards us, are for good and not for evil, to give us a future and a hope. (Jeremiah 29:11). There is lots more!

Prayer is sometimes misunderstood. Some think we pray once and then make a 'faith stand.' But the scripture is clear, 'Ask and it will be given you,' and *'For everyone who asks receives.'* (Matthew 7:7-8)
The important point is that 'ask' is in the present tense.
 In Greek the present tense is, unlike English, reserved for current continuing action – *'For everyone who is asking receives,'* not a one off event.

[In Greek the present tense is not used for past action - that is the imperfect tense.]

Why doesn't God just answer a simple request to have anxiety taken away? Maybe sometimes He does! However, what 'we think' is the main driver of anxiety and what 'we think' is in the realm of our free will. If we choose to think these negative things – well He will let us do so. The bottom line is our choice.

The sufferer from acute anxiety needs help to recognise the problem and to be encouraged into dealing with the falsehoods he or she sees as reality, though they are just paper tigers.

The role of prayer is to be much more specific. That is to deal with parts of the problem bit by bit rather than a sweeping 'Take it away, Lord.'

For example of prayer for a specific part of anxiety: Sleeping well is very important to our wellbeing. For the sufferer from anxiety sleep can be interrupted or disturbed by unconscious 'red' or bad thoughts. The born again believer can pray to the indwelling Holy Spirit before sleeping, asking Him to be a doorkeeper over his or her mind and emotions, preventing these unconscious thoughts entering during the night hours.

Listen for help and hope

The Lord God will help and will answer prayer – we need to listen. The Holy Spirit will bring words and scriptures and pictures to mind in response to our prayers.

His words and pictures are very encouraging and they prove that we are not alone as we journey through all of life, its pitfalls and specifically through anxiety.

Furthermore the Lord God knows exactly what will help us at any given time – an encouraging word, an encouraging scripture, a picture. Things which bring hope.

So whilst He doesn't usually just sweep away anxiety, we do find, just like Paul, that His grace and mercy are sufficient. (2 Corinthians 12:9)

Chapter 6 – notes

Important Points

Pray bit by bit for help with individual aspects of the problem - you will see results. Listen for the Holy Spirit.

Your notes -

Chapter 7
Free and staying free - the biblical perspective.

This chapter describes what the bible says for those who believe and are born again by the Spirit of God.

Freedom   Scripture tells us that there are two sources of freedom for us.
'Therefore if the Son makes you free (and He certainly does) you shall be free indeed.'
John 8:36
'And you shall know the truth and the truth will set you free'. John 8:32
Born again you have been set free.

World ruler   There is a spiritual world ruler. Jesus called him the *'prince of this world'* and *'the ruler of this world.'* John 12:31 and 14:30

Lies   The world ruler, whose is known as satan or the devil, is a liar. Jesus tells us that, before we become born again, we are of our father the devil and that he is a murderer and liar because there is no truth in him. John 8:44

Born again   It is for this reason Jesus said we must be born again – otherwise we cannot see the Kingdom of Heaven. John 3:3. This is to be understood literally. Our human spirit which was dead through sin at the fall of man (we died in Adam), is literally born again with God now the literal Father of our human spirit. We have a new Father!

Stand	Born again - Then we are advised of the need to stand against the wiles (schemes) of the enemy Ephesians 6:11
Reality	There are hosts of evil spiritual beings set against us – these are enemies of God and of us. Ephesians 6:12 To a significant degree we can be in denial of this reality and need to change our thinking. Evil spiritual beings are real and active and present here, spreading evil as we can easily see is prolific in the world around us.
Anxiety	*'Be anxious for nothing.'* Philippians 4:6

Here is the problem for the one suffering from anxiety:

Anxiety is unreasonable uneasiness. When acute it is very painful and dangerous sometimes leading even to suicide. Anxiety is about what might or might not happen in the future, whether that is the immediate future, a bit later or more long term. It has the appearance of being absolute reality to the sufferer. However in reality it is lies and comes from the father of lies – our and God's enemy. The bible believing sufferer is then subject to the difficulty of thoughts that appear very real – once he or she knows, or is easily shown, that his or her anxiety is irrational; and knows that the bible says, *'do not be anxious,'* he or she has a problem! – How to move on from anxiety to freedom.

Be certain of the objective. Freedom from anxiety is fully available. That does not mean there will never ever be an anxious thought. It means that, in the same way as one not suffering from anxiety can easily brush aside these lies of the enemy, so in like manner it will become the same for you.

Then, certain of the objective, follow the way to peace.

Peace   Jesus said, *'Peace I leave with you, My peace I give to you, not as the world gives do I give to you. Let not your heart be troubled, neither let it be afraid.'* John 14:27

Mind renewal   Paper tigers, anxious thoughts, are arguments from the devil, setting themselves against the truth – and thus against the knowledge of God. So we are advised in scripture:
'Though we walk in the flesh, we do not war according to the flesh. For the weapons of our warfare are not carnal but mighty in God for pulling down strongholds, casting down arguments and every high thing (or pretension) that exalts itself against the knowledge of God, bringing every thought into captivity to the obedience of Christ' 2 Corinthians 10:3-5 And ....

'And do not be conformed to this world, but be transformed by the renewing of your mind, that you may prove what is that good and acceptable and perfect will of God.' Romans 12:2

Apply   Anxiety is the fruit of believing what is
             fed into our minds by the evil forces of the ruler
             of this world, by others, or even by our own flesh.
             It appears like reality, but anxiety is only lies. In
             the 1960's and 70's there was fear of a nuclear
             world war. The fear was irrational.
             If there had been a nuclear world war could
             you or I have done anything about it? No!
             However the anxiety was just lies and
             speculation – there was no nuclear world
             war. All anxiety was pointless.

Pray   Seek help from the Lord. It is likely to be difficult
         to apply the self helps we have outlined. It does
         need to be worked at. (That is why typically a
         course of Cognitive Behavioural Therapy
         will take many weeks. Prayer will help – ask for
         help in any and every area of difficulty in believing
         and in applying the truth.

Persevere   Keep in mind the objective. Remember the
            promise. Psalm 23 has, *'though I walk through the
            valley of the shadow of death (and it can seem like
            that) I will fear no evil for You are with me and
            Your rod and staff they comfort me. You prepare a
            table for me in the presence of my enemies. You
            anoint my head with oil, my cup runs over. Surely
            goodness and mercy shall follow me all the days of my
            life and I will dwell in the house of the Lord forever.'*

            Keep the Lord always before you and always in
            your mind. He is the answer, not the problem.
            Speak with Him - often.

Staying free is a matter of continuing in the revelation that anxiety is the work of our enemy and keeping ourselves free of 'red' or bad thoughts by the renewing of our minds.

Strongholds

It is possible that a stronghold may have developed. It will be recognised, not necessarily by the sufferer, but by others close to them. When a stronghold has developed the sufferer will not even be able to think straight for periods of time.
See 'Demolishing strongholds – dealing with intractable problems.' (Available on Amazon or on freebiblebooklets.com)

Evil Spirits

A lot of Jesus ministry on earth was dealing with, casting out evil spirits. This can be necessary for sufferers from anxiety, but is not necessarily needed. Discernment definitely is needed. Prayer seeking discernment will certainly be appropriate. Then act according to the discernment given to you by God.
Evil spirits are not able to prevent you from coming to Jesus. Even legion could not prevent the demoniac from falling at Jesus feet. Nevertheless the full release for him came when legion was dismissed. (Luke 8:26-39)

Casting out a spirit(s) from a sufferer of anxiety, when shown that this is appropriate by the Lord, will be very significant in their recovery. But timing will be very important. The sufferer needs to be in a position of calm and not in a high state of anxiety for freedom to be accomplished – otherwise, in a high state of anxiety false manifestations which look like spirits being expelled can be produced causing disillusionment. Be certain to seek the Holy Spirit regarding timing!

In the meantime applying the self-helps will produce a lot of benefit.

Chapter 7 – Notes

Important points

The bible is the word of truth 'breathed' by God through the writers, to make us complete and to thoroughly equip us for every good work. (2 Timothy 3:17)

Your notes

Appendix
What anxiety can be like by one who has suffered it.

Once in negative thought mode, it's like a magnet drawing in many other negative thoughts.

The pattern of these thoughts present a reality, they feel true. Because of this it is very difficult to fully recognise the true reality. Often one needs the help of another to enable the individual to recognise the 'true' reality.

At times it is literally like a filter is in place. You can hear the truth and give mental ascent to what you are hearing being correct but it is as though the truth is not able to penetrate the filter in order to bring about the difference.

Not always easy to recognise the lies for what they are such as 'You will never be free of this'

The longer this type of thought pattern, which is the root of the anxiety, has continued the harder it is, and the more effort that is required to come into correct thinking.

There is nearly always, if not always, a trigger for the anxiety / panic. It isn't always easy to identify the trigger but there will be one. Once it is found it becomes much easier to realise the wrong thinking that is taking place.

One practical way of gaining some relief is to engage in an activity which demands concentration - as this puts the mind onto something else such as photography, music, completing a puzzle etc.

When the thoughts are intense causing anxiety it can also result in physical pains such as the feeling of the stomach being held in a tight fist, or making it harder to eat without some form of discomfort.

Can be extremely helpful to picture a pirate's large sturdy chest with a padlock on. In your 'mind's eye' open the chest, one by one put in the disturbing thoughts, close the lid and close the padlock.

When the anxiety is really bad it can make you feel as though you are very much alone in it. On the one hand you know that this is not the case but it very much feels that way. There is the feeling that no one will really understand what is happening.

Again at times of intensity it can feel as though you are not connecting with the world, as though somehow you are cut off from it. This can feel quite frightening.

During times of anxiety caused by negative thinking it often feels as though the mind is on overdrive, constantly active jumping from one thing to another.
Concentration can become more difficult as a result of the above.

There can be a real sense of frustration with oneself because on the one hand you know much of it is irrational but on the other hand there is the feeling of being powerless to do anything about it. Thoughts such as 'Why can't I deal with this', 'What's wrong with me' 'No one else will really understand what is going on' etc etc these often present themselves.

Giving the degree of intensity a score from 0 -10 can be extremely helpful. For instance if the score in the morning is 8 and in the afternoon is 7 then in the evening is 6 there is tremendous encouragement to know that even though things are still fairly intense at least things are getting easier therefore confirming 'I will get out of this

Other titles:
The ICCC – Transformed Working Life series:
Inherent Power
Work is a 1st class calling
No one can serve two masters
Hope - the certainty of future blessing
Faith or presumption
Hearing God speak
Working from rest
Renewing the mind
Be strong in the battle
Anointing
Fruitfulness
Other booklets written for ICCC
Powered by grace
Works of power - now is the time
Stand tall - take your position
Transformed Working Life - quick view
Inspiration from word for the week - 1 to 52
Inspiration from word for the week - 53 to 104
Inspiration from word for the week -105-156

Other publications
Will the church be caught away?
Explaining the future.
Rightly dividing the word of truth.
So that's what it's all about   (overview of the bible account)
*Daniel (introductory level)
*Revelation (introductory level)
Ostrich Christianity
Israel and the church not in competition

Favour - enjoying the children's bread.
What should we do with money?
Going for Gold – the testing and stretching of our faith
After Brexit – the nature of the battle ahead
Last Orders
Wisdom
The King is coming
Health and Healing
The sign of Jonah – solved
Understanding the parable of the 10 virgins
The Kingdom Way
The Persistent Widow
Can I lose my salvation?
Meet the Teacher
Love, 153 fish and seven signs
Paul's thorn in the flesh - its message for today
Deception and how to avoid it
Chosen and Choice
The end is not quite yet
Amazing numbers
Blood – the blood of the New Covenant
Building spiritual strength
Grace and judgement
The believer's authority
God's eternal purpose
And God spoke - hearing God speak today
Understanding Hebrews
Reigning in life
Inspiration from Word for the week
Jesus said Watch
Creation? Evolution? Difficult to choose.
Made in God's image – why and what does it mean
Grace and peace from the seven spirits

James and the meaning of faith
The story of time
Is the bible reliable?
The way of the moon
Practical spiritual warfare
Parables
Jesus pathway through life
Sons, Children, servants
The fear of God and the love of God
Keep your heart with all diligence
Demolishing strongholds

To access printed copies at Amazon - type peter michell in the search box.

* Not in print

All booklets are available as free PDF downloads at www.freebiblebooklets.com

Printed in Great Britain
by Amazon